BIOIDENTICAL HORMONES:

HELL OR HEAVEN?

HOW BIOIDENTICAL HORMONES CAN GIVE YOU SUPPORT TO HELP IMPROVE YOUR HEALTH AND OVERALL WELL-BEING

SERGEY KALITENKO, MD

authorHOUSE®

AuthorHouse™
1663 Liberty Drive
Bloomington, IN 47403
www.authorhouse.com
Phone: 1 (800) 839-8640

Published by AuthorHouse   08/26/2016

ISBN: 978-1-5246-2633-4 (sc)
ISBN: 978-1-5246-2632-7 (e)

Library of Congress Control Number: 2016914012

Print information available on the last page.

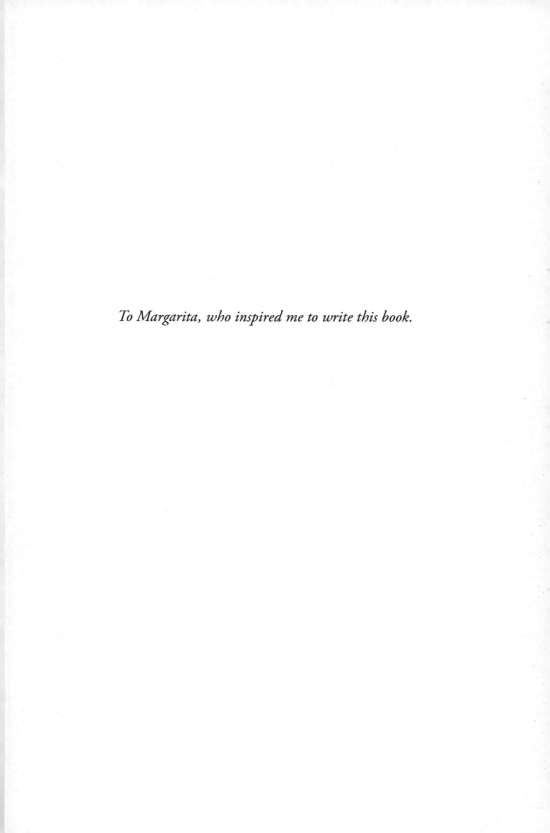

To Margarita, who inspired me to write this book.

Contents

Introduction

"Life-threatening heart problems don't necessary originate from the heart itself. The problem could be in a totally different place," said the emergency room doctor.

Several of my colleagues and I were having lunch in the hospital cafeteria.

"If you're talking about infection or inflammation, you're not telling me anything new," I said.

"Far from it. I'm talking about a much bigger problem that is often overlooked. And in my opinion, being aware of this can save lives."

"What do you mean? Please explain."

"This morning, a middle-aged woman—let's call her Susan—came to the emergency room because of shortness of breath. It was so bad that she had almost passed out and fallen down. Fortunately, the ambulance came quickly and brought her here. According to her husband, Susan was healthy before. When she came in, she was pale and looked anxious. There was fear in her eyes. Fear of death. Her blood pressure was low, and her pulse was irregular."

"This is nothing unusual. You were most likely dealing with acute heart attack complicated by irregular heartbeats with possible cardiogenic shock. Did you transfer her to a cardiology intensive care unit?"

"Not at all."

"Why not?"

"Because Susan didn't have a heart attack. I considered a heart attack from the beginning and managed her accordingly. But we needed a confirmation—cardiac enzymes. In the computer, they were still pending. So I called the lab. 'How about enzymes?' I asked. The technician replied, 'Wait a second. I'll take a look.' These seconds felt like hours. Finally the lab technician stated, 'Negative.' I did not know what to do. Susan still might have a heart attack because it might take hours for enzymes to show up in the blood. So was it still a heart attack or it was something else?

"If it was a heart attack, she'd require one type of management. If it wasn't a heart attack, then she'd require a totally different management approach. I was thinking about other causes for her irregular heartbeats—atrial fibrillation. Could it be lack of oxygen? I called the respiratory tech to check Susan's arterial blood gases. A few minutes later, the report came back normal. Could it be alcohol withdrawal? I called her husband. 'Is your wife a heavy drinker?'

"'Not at all—in fact, she doesn't drink alcohol at all.'

"'How about coffee?'

"'No, Doc—maybe a cup on a weekend, but not always.'

"I was running out of possibilities. High blood sugar? I checked Susan's biochemistry profile. Normal. Structural heart problem like mitral valve stenosis? How could I have missed this from the beginning? I grabbed a phone to call an ultrasound technician. 'I need ECHO stat in ER.' In a few minutes, the tech arrived with a portable ultrasound machine. She plugged it in, put a gel on the patient's chest, and started scanning. I watched, trying to get an answer as soon as possible.

"'So? Did you find anything?' I asked.

"'Doc,' the tech answered, taking a deep breath. 'She has a gorgeous heart. No structural problems at all.'

"I started losing hope. What else could it be? I was running out of possibilities and running out of time. Susan's blood pressure kept dropping. I decided to do cardioversion to restore normal heart rhythm. We charged the defibrillator. Fifty joules—charged. I put the pads on her chest. Everybody's clear? Shock. Her body jumped. A quick look at the heart monitor—nothing. Still in atrial fibrillation. Charging again. Now 100 joules. Everybody's clear? Shock. Her body jumped again. Heart monitor—still in atrial fibrillation. Now 200 joules. Is everybody clear? Shock. Everybody's jumping. Cardiac monitor—no change. We failed.

"The only thing that was left was to give Susan oxygen and IV fluids. I was desperate. Were we missing something? I was desperately looking for possible causes of her heart problem. I knew that if we didn't figure out what was going on with her, we'd lose her. The clock was ticking. Susan's husband came to the nursing station.

"'How is my wife doing, Doc?' he asked.

"'No good news yet, I'm afraid. Your wife's condition is unstable, and we're still investigating what is going on.'

"'I know that you're doing everything you can, Doc. But I forgot to tell you that Susan was complaining about some discomfort around her throat.' And he showed me where—around his Adam's apple. 'Is this the thyroid gland, Doc?'

"*Oh my God*, I thought. *Of course, it's her thyroid gland!* I rushed to the phone to call the lab. 'I need to back order a thyroid profile on this patient. When do I need it? As soon as possible.'

"Twenty minutes later, they paged me overhead. 'ER doctor, please call the lab stat.' I jumped to the phone and almost ripped the receiver off the wall. 'What is it?' 'Her TSH is almost undetectable, and her T3 and T4 are sky-high,' said the technician. I took a deep breath. It was not a heart attack. It was hyperthyroidism; that's what was causing her atrial fibrillation. We immediately took the appropriate actions. And Susan started getting better. Her life was saved."

"I think you're right," said the cardiologist, who along with the rest of us had remained silent up to this point. "I always take a patient's hormonal status into consideration. For example, if a woman comes to the emergency room with chest pain, the first question I ask is, "Do you still have monthly periods?" Because if a woman is still menstruating, her sex hormones like estrogen, progesterone, and testosterone will be up, and her risk for heart disease will be low. But if she no longer has periods, her hormones will be down. Her risk for heart disease will be high, and she'll need an extensive workup."

"I'll tell you more," added the orthopedic doctor, now ready to share his thoughts as well. "Today I have a couple of women scheduled for surgery because of hip fracture. As you know, hip fracture might be a life-threatening condition. Why do women have hip fractures? Because of osteoporosis. But what is the reason for osteoporosis? Lack of hormones, mainly estrogen. So if, God forbid, one of those women dies, they'll attribute it to hip fracture. But she may have actually died due to lack of hormones—and because she was never put on bioidentical hormone replacement therapy. Unfortunately, nobody links hip fracture to lack of hormones."

"It's the same thing with a heart attack," chimed in the cardiologist. "If a woman dies because of a heart attack or cancer, we blame cholesterol, cancer cells, or genes. But nobody links cancer or heart failure to a lack of hormones. When a woman is young and her hormone levels are high, she usually doesn't have a heart attack or cancer or high blood pressure. It's when she goes into menopause and her hormones go all the way down that the problems start."

1. How a Big Disaster Begins

You're in your forties or fifties. You have everything you've ever dreamed of: a wonderful spouse, beautiful kids, and a rewarding job or business. Everything is going smoothly, and you think that it's finally time to relax and enjoy life.

Suddenly you feel like you're on fire. You turn red and start sweating. It can happen at the most inopportune times, like while you're in bed with your loved one or speaking to one of your customers. After a few minutes, the hot flash is gone, but it comes back again and again. What's going on?

Then you start noticing other things. You forget appointments or where you left your keys, and you need to make a shopping list so you remember everything you need at the store. You have mood swings and yell at your children and spouse for no reason. Quality sleep is elusive, and you pass up invitations to go out with friends because you're tired. Sex has become routine, not enjoyable, and even painful, but avoiding it causes further problems. And when you look in the mirror, you see wrinkles that you swear weren't there the day before. One after another, the autopilots in your life shut off, and things don't seem easy anymore.

Going through menopause or andropause can be like trying to cross a stormy Atlantic Ocean in a rowboat. You feel like you're being sucked into the waves of despair without any means of rescue. You're crying out for help, but the life you worked so hard to get is now sinking.

2. The Position of Official Medicine

You visit your primary care physician and then your psychiatrist—to no avail. No one is able to explain why you're suffering and what needs to be done to alleviate it. To your frustration, your doctor attributes it to aging, which is normal. However, you know something is seriously wrong—and that if left untreated, it will continue to cause you physical and mental anguish.

Could there be one simple test that can prevent such a disaster?

Official Western medicine does not have an answer to this question. According to demographer S. Jay Olshansky of the University of Illinois (as well as fifty-one longevity experts in their position statement in 2002), nothing can be done to prolong life significantly. Isn't it sad?

3. A Common-Sense Perspective

Because of this, I launched my own investigation.

My investigation was based on facts and common sense, not controlled studies. Dr. James Lind successfully used this method in the 1700s when he discovered how to fight scurvy. Six groups of two sailors were used, and the group that was given oranges and lemons actually improved. Dr. Edward Jenner used this same method in 1796 when he invented the vaccination for smallpox.

What would happen to mankind if double-blind, controlled studies were necessary to prove that the vaccination works for smallpox, or lemon for scurvy? We would be dead. If a treatment is really working, you don't need double-blind, controlled studies to prove it.

It's like the key for your front door. It either fits or it doesn't.

4. Synthetic Hormones: Salvation or Frustration?

Large studies are typically conducted by groups of scientists and financed by even larger pharmaceutical companies. Such was the case in funding research to create drugs that mimic human hormones.

Since natural substances like hormones cannot be patented, scientists had to come up with alternatives. Instead of offering estrogen (the most important woman's hormone), they provided modified horse estrogens to produce synthetic estrogen for women. And instead of offering progesterone, the second-most important women's hormone, they furnished progestins—which sound remarkably like natural progesterone but are actually synthetic.

In the beginning, everybody was happy: patients, because they felt better; doctors, because it was less work for them; and pharmaceutical companies, because they were making money.

Until the Women's Health Initiative (WHI) study came out.

Synthetic and semisynthetic drugs such as Premarin and Prempro that mimicked hormones were the crown jewels of pharmaceutical companies. Their sales reached almost one billion dollars in 2001.[1] However, even Big Pharma couldn't conceal the WHI study's damaging conclusions that these synthetic or semisynthetic hormones were linked to many life-threatening conditions like cancer and blood clots.

But these drugs were on the market already and had proven to be very profitable. What the pharmaceutical companies had to do was warn patients about the inherent risks while continuing to sell the drugs to maintain their cash flows. But why did the FDA approve drugs that had potentially life-threatening side effects in the first place?

In 2009, *New York Times* reporter Natasha Singer looked into hormone replacement therapy drugs. She wasn't interested in how those drugs were approved after the scandals with Troglitazone[2] or Trovan[3] but rather was intrigued by something much more important—how it happened that doctors recommended harmful drugs. What she found was that ghostwritten medical papers, signed by doctors, had created a medical "consensus." [4]

5. Can We Trust Such "Scientific" Articles?

I still remember my twenty-seven-year-old neighbor who was on birth control pills and died from a blood clot in her legs that traveled into her lungs. It was because of that, as well as the following factors, that I decided not to advise traditional synthetic or semisynthetic hormones for my patients:

- They are linked to cancer.[5]
- They can cause blood clots.[6]

- Low testosterone, decreased libido, and gallstones are linked to the use of synthetic hormones.[7]

But do you need hormones at all? Maybe you can get your life back with diet and supplements. Or maybe all you need to do is bring your cholesterol down. What about yoga and meditation?

When I started practicing, one of my first patients suffered from a heart attack. He was gasping, in a cold sweat, with fear in his eyes and death imprinted on his face. Another of my patients was in excruciating pain from cancer. Alzheimer's patients know about their problem and are ashamed of it. Could I offer them meditation and yoga as a solution of their problems? Traditional medicine would suggest that maybe all we need to do is get heart, cancer, and dementia treatments. But do they really work?

6. Why Eskimos Don't Have Heart Attacks

During my medical training, I was told many times that heart attacks were due to high cholesterol. What I didn't know about then was the Danish Eskimo study.[8]

Danish scientists Bang and Dyerberg discovered that Eskimos almost never had heart attacks, the US number-one killer, despite the fact that they don't have very low cholesterol. So it wasn't actually cholesterol that kills, and they had known about this since the 1970s! It must be something else. What about cancer? What about Alzheimer's?

Staffan Lindeberg, MD, a Swedish scientist from the University of Lund, went to the Kitava Island in New Guinea to study its population of 24,000 inhabitants. He found that they didn't have heart attacks either! Or cancer! No diabetes! No Alzheimer's! However, they die healthy, on average, at the age of forty-five mainly because of high infant and childhood mortality.[9] If they survive childhood, they live a long life and die in their eighties or nineties.

So if it isn't cholesterol, cancer, or dementia that kills, what is it? I was at a dead end, and there was no help in sight. Do you think that

Big Pharma will give away money to figure out a way to help you get better naturally?

Seeing is believing. Have you ever seen a person who looks half as young as her real age? She has beautiful skin and bright eyes. Her dress cannot conceal the gorgeous curves of her body, and her voice reaches to the bottom of everybody's heart. She looks like she's in her early thirties, but she is, in fact, in her sixties. Her name is Suzanne Somers, and her "fountain of youth" is bioidentical hormone replacement.

So what is she doing right? Maybe her thought is correct that it isn't your cholesterol, and it isn't your blood pressure; it's the decline of hormones that kills you?

Really? What about heart attacks, cancer, and Alzheimer's?

If you develop a chest pain in your twenties, it's usually a pulled muscle (not always). But if you experience chest pain in your seventies, it's most likely a heart attack.

We usually don't have heart attacks, Alzheimer's, or cancer in our twenties when our sex hormone levels are high, but we do have them when our sex hormones are down.

Why?

Quite simply, because Mother Nature doesn't have much use for us once we can't make babies anymore, and we need to free space for younger individuals who can. There is almost no menopause or andropause in the animal kingdom unless the animal is in captivity and consuming unnatural foods. But fortunately for us, there is a loophole for humans—menopause and andropause—that ensures humans are superior in survival compared to any other species in the world.

7. The Meaning of Menopause and Andropause

A pleasant, middle-aged woman sat in my office with tears rolling down her face. Her boyfriend had threatened to leave her because of her vaginal dryness and night sweats. She went to her primary-care physician but was told her symptoms were a normal reaction to menopause. However, this didn't make her boyfriend change his mind. She needed help right away.

Normally, a fertile woman's ovaries have plenty of eggs that are released in cycles. In order to get pregnant at the beginning of her menstrual cycle, she produces the sex hormone estrogen, which makes the egg-laden follicles grow. When the egg is big enough, follicle-stimulating hormones and luteinizing hormones surge, which along with estrogen makes the follicle break—a process called ovulation.

Ovaries then start producing another sex hormone, progesterone. The freed egg travels to the progesterone-prepared uterus. If there is sperm there, pregnancy commences. If not, the egg is released, the production of estrogen and progesterone ceases, the uterus lining goes, blood vessels open, and menstrual bleeding starts. Estrogen production resumes, the uterus lining is restored, the bleeding is over, and a woman is ready for another cycle. These cycles continue until there are no more eggs in a woman's ovaries. When there are no more eggs, periods stop and menopause begins. Sounds simple. But there is a problem here: an average woman has about one million eggs, yet she uses only about four hundred in her reproductive years. Same thing with men: when testicular biopsies were performed on elderly men, they found many unused spermatozoids. Why?

According to the Bible, Adam lived for 930 years, and many people believe that Eve lived for approximately six hundred years. Maybe that's why men and women have so many spermatozoon and eggs—we're supposed to live for centuries. But if that's the case, shouldn't we be able to procreate longer? Why are these seemingly valuable eggs and sperm being wasted?

Maybe Mother Nature wants a postmenopausal woman to take care of her daughter's children so that she can make more babies. This is what the grandmother theory states.[10] Or maybe it's because older males can compete with youngsters because older males are more experienced and sophisticated. This is what the patriarch hypothesis says.[11]

Something else to consider is what's known as the "cortisol steal." Estrogen, progesterone, and testosterone are made from cholesterol, the same precursor as the anti-inflammatory hormone cortisol. But the amount of cholesterol in the body is limited. So when the body is experiencing chronic inflammation, it has to decide which it needs more: cortisol, to keep the inflammation under control, or sex hormones. Since the body perceives the inflammation as life-threatening, it opts for the cortisol—essentially "stealing" the cholesterol from producing estrogen, progesterone, and testosterone, which causes the symptoms associated with menopause and andropause, such as low libido, painful sexual intercourse, insufficient vaginal lubrication, and difficulty maintaining erections.

What if the solution for menopause was as simple as removing the source of the inflammation?

When it comes down to it, it doesn't matter why we were given menopause and andropause; what matters is that we might have a loophole to get our lives back. The only thing we need to do is to trick our bodies into believing that we're still young. But how?

8. How to Pretend to Be Young

A middle-aged man sitting in my office said desperately, "Doc, help me! I need to get this thing up now!"

"Why it is so urgent?" I asked.

"Because she's much younger than me," said the man. I tried to explain that a man in his fifties can't expect to perform the same as an eighteen-year-old man. He refused to listen. "I love her, Doc; I can't make her unhappy because I can't perform. I can't lose her, because if I do, I will die without her." What could I have told him? That he shouldn't have married a young girl? I couldn't say that because love knows nothing about age. I needed to help him now. And I had something in mind regarding how to do it.

In 1930, a young chairman in the Department of Biochemistry at McGill University, Professor Dr. James Collip, had just codiscovered insulin and was thinking about how to get relief from menopausal ailments. After a series of experiments and failures, he eventually found the solution by extracting estrogen from the urine of pregnant women and providing it as a menopausal remedy. Giving natural hormones of fertile women to postmenopausal individuals sent a signal to their bodies that they were still fertile. That's how we can pretend we're still young.

Have you ever run out of gas? Certainly. But you didn't think that it was the end of the world or that your car wouldn't run anymore. What you did was go to a gas station and fill up the tank, right?

The same line of thinking applies here. If you run out of eggs or sperm, you simply need to fill your body with hormones that are exactly the same as your own. But which hormones exactly are we talking about here? Mainly estrogen, progesterone, and testosterone.

Have you ever seen a picture of Marilyn Monroe? She's the perfect example of a woman who is full of estrogen: confident and big-breasted, with a strong desire to have sex and a low waist-to-hip ratio.[12] That's why estrogen is sometimes called the "Marilyn Monroe Hormone."

Estrogen plays a critical role in a human's body. It is responsible for skin and blood vessels, breast development, vaginal lubrication, fat burning, and bone and cholesterol maintenance. Since it works as an antioxidant, it is linked to your brain protection. Lack of estrogen is linked to mood problems[13] and memory problems. However, estrogen alone is not enough.

Confidence and strong sexual desire should be balanced; otherwise, they will go too far. The hormone that does the job is progesterone.

Have you ever noticed how calm most pregnant women are? It's because of the presence of progesterone. And if you drink a glass of milk before bed to get better sleep, the progesterone from milk is probably helping you relax. Milk also contains calcium and the milk protein casein, which, when broken down into casomorphin in your stomach, is an opioid[14] (almost like a street drug).

Of course the progesterone your body produces is not morphine, but it balances estrogen, calms you down, normalizes blood pressure, and works as a natural diuretic and antidepressant. Not just a sex hormone, progesterone is also a neuro-steroid that is produced in your brain and is necessary for normal brain function.

But again, estrogen and progesterone are not enough. There needs to be something that gives us energy and a sense of well-being, as well as the ability to maintain our muscles, mental strength, and libido. That's where testosterone comes in.

In 1889, Doctor Charles-Edouard Brown-Sequard—a former Harvard professor and current professor of experimental medicine at College de France—sought an elixir of youth. He was a shrewd observer and talented scientist, and his name is immortalized in modern neurology by the eponymous spinal cord damage syndrome. But he was getting old like everyone else and was desperately looking for an antiaging remedy. After self-administered injections of an extract from guinea pigs testicles, his vigor and well-being returned. His elixir—later called the Brown-Séquard Elixir—was testosterone, and his observations were first published in the *Lancet* medical journal.

While his colleagues initially laughed at him, forty years later the importance of testosterone was rediscovered.[15] Now we know that testosterone made in your body doesn't just linked to benefiting the sex drive, erections, and muscles but also linked to maintaining bones and protecting you from diabetes, Alzheimer's, and heart disease.[16]

The bottom line is men and women need all three hormones— estrogen, progesterone, and testosterone—to get the support they need to truly benefit.

9. Are Bioidentical Hormones Officially Recommended?'

When a drug company representative (we call them "drug dealers") came to my office selling some prescription drugs, I asked him, "Do you have bioidentical hormones?" He said, "Nope." I asked why. He answered, "Doc, don't you know that according to American laws, natural substances can't be patented? No patent, no money!"

No other treatment has ignited as many debates and controversy as bioidentical hormone replacement therapy (BHRT). Medical institutions, including the FDA, International Menopause Society, American Medical Association, Endocrine Society, Mayo Clinic, and the American College of Obstetricians and Gynecologists, have stated that bioidentical hormones carry the same risks as synthetic hormones and that there is no evidence of any additional benefits.

Why is there such a perfect consensus about it? Recently, two branches of government research tried to decide if chronic fatigue syndrome was associated with the exotic XMRV virus. One group (Harvey Alter, FDA and National Institutes of Health) found that there was a link. Another group (William Switzer, CDC) found the contrary.[17]

If scientists who are using the same methods and tests on the same virus can't come to the same conclusion, how could they be so unanimous on a more complicated subject like bioidentical hormones?

As for the FDA's decision that the risks of bioidenticals are the same as those for synthetic hormones, what are these opinions based on? Did the FDA test bioidentical hormones? Not that I'm aware of. They assumed that bioidenticals work the same as synthetic hormones—which we know might be, in fact, harmful. It's like assuming that a one-dollar bill has the same value as a hundred-dollar bill, because they're the same size.

On the other hand, proponents of bioidentical hormone replacement therapy are saying that these hormones are safe and have almost no side effects.

Two French studies published in 2008 suggest that bioidenticals are safer than conventional HRT. According to Dr. Kent Holtorf's literature review, bioidentical hormones appear to be safer and more potent then synthetic versions. Therefore, physicians may opt for bioidenticals for now unless new data is available from new studies.[18]

Even some prominent clinicians have to publicly admit the advantages of bioidenticals.

According to Dr. Christine Derzko, chief of endocrinology at St. Michael's Hospital in Toronto, although it is too early to say for sure, bioidentical hormones carry at least the same but sometimes less risk than synthetic hormones.[19]

Normally, we'd need controlled randomized studies of the efficacy and safety of bioidentical hormones, but there is no such study in sight.

Do you think Big Pharma will invest money in something that can't be patented and therefore is unlikely to be profitable?

But what do we do if we lack long-term studies so far? Let's see what experts say. According to Professor Leon Speroff, if a physician doesn't have clear-cut evidence, he might consider giving the treatment the patient prefers because there is no guarantee that appropriate clinical trials will be done in the near future (*Clinical Gynecologic Endocrinology and Infertility*). Dr. Speroff is a professor of obstetrics and gynecology at Oregon Health and Science University and a subspecialist in reproductive endocrinology. One of the most respected OB/GYN doctors in the country, he's also the founder and recent director for the Women's Health Research Unit at OHSU. He has gained prominence in the area of women's health throughout his publications, national and international lectures, and extensive work on clinical trials.

But do bioidentical hormones really work? Do they really prolong life? Or are they just another myth?

10. How Longevity Secrets Were Revealed

Another breakthrough came unexpectedly—from the Blue Zones study.

Because official medicine and traditional doctors don't offer a longevity prescription, *National Geographic* reporter Dan Buettner decided to look for the areas on earth where people lived longer than other populations. After studying people in key Blue Zone areas (Sardinia, Italy; Okinawa, Japan; Loma Linda, California, US; and Nicoya, Costa Rica), he and his team learned the following life-enhancing lessons:

- Get enough exposure to the sun.
- Eat nuts and tomatoes.
- Be social.
- Restrict your caloric consumption.
- Move naturally.
- Drink enough water.

Doesn't sound unusual, but somehow together they worked much better than any other recommended protocol. What was the secret behind the Blue Zones' lessons?

The solution came unexpectedly. While investigating the benefits of tomatoes, recommended by Blue Zones' conclusions, I learned that the most valuable of their components, the antioxidant lycopene, goes to the testes, adrenal glands, and liver. It seemed like tomatoes might be protecting endocrine glands from oxidative stress, but for what? To make sure that they make enough hormones! I thought to myself, *Maybe it is all about hormones!*

Being social means less stress and hence less of the harmful cortisol—and more of the other steroids like estrogen, progesterone, and testosterone. Caloric restriction is linked to raised human growth hormone (HGH) levels. Sun exposure provides vitamin D, which is considered more as a hormone now.

Forget for a second about Blue Zones. The longest-living person on earth is Jeanne Calment, who lived for 122 years and 165 days. She was riding a bicycle at age one hundred and broke her hip at age 114. This means that she had enough estrogen to maintain her bones! Another centenarian, Rafael Angel Leon from Nicoya, had multiple girlfriends until age ninety-four and then married a woman who was forty years younger than he was!

So if longevity is all about hormones, how about safety?

11. Are Bioidentical Hormones Safe?

It's like trying to answer the question if drinking water is safe. Yes, drinking water is safe but in moderation. If you drink too much, your brain will swell to the extent that you may die.

Because bioidentical hormones are structurally identical to your own hormones, many doctors opt for bioidenticals rather than synthetic hormones. Many patients also opt for bioidenticals because of the same reason. However, in my opinion, hormones—even bioidenticals—are still hormones. This is much more complicated than just comparing bioidentical and synthetic hormones.

Obviously, estrogen itself is not a problem, because your body cannot produce a poisonous hormone. The problem comes when there is too much estrogen, which might lead to an increased cancer risk. Or estrogen is converted into a poison that causes cancer.

Normally, the main body estrogen—estradiol or E2—is removed from your body very rapidly:

1. It is converted into 2 OH estrone, which is benign.
2. It binds to bile in the stomach, becomes water soluble, and is then eliminated via the kidneys.

However, three conditions are required for the removal of estradiol:

1. Your body knows what to do with the hormone.
2. There are enough enzymes to do the job.
3. Your digestive system functions properly and does not have too much bad bacteria in it.

If even a single condition isn't met, you may be in danger.

Unlike bioidenticals, your body doesn't know that to do with synthetic and semisynthetic estrogens. Therefore, isn't it possible that instead of 2 OH estrone, they might be transformed more than usual into 4 OH estrone—which can lead to free radical formation and hence cancer?

I assume, bioidenticals don't have this problem if your body is functioning properly, but what if your body doesn't have enough enzymes? Or your stomach isn't functioning properly? Then the same story—bioidentical hormones are transformed into 4 OH estrone that might lead to free radical formation and subsequently cancer. Or they are not eliminated properly and start piling up in your body, creating estrogen dominance.

Fortunately, we can monitor what your body is doing with estrogen as well as its level and, most of the time, correct it.

12. The Bottom Line Is Simple

Get more energy, better sleep, and improved mood, productivity, and sex life with the support of bioidentical hormone replacement therapy (BHRT). Many doctors believe that BHRT is very effective and reasonably safe, but as with any health regimen, you need to be aware of the risks involved.

If your doctor determines that BHRT may be an appropriate option for you, you might benefit from complementing your hormone therapy with a well-balanced, organic diet. You've heard the saying, "You are what you eat," and all indications are that the higher the quality of food that you consume, the better your body might perform with the support of quality food. Not only that, but your mind will be sharper, and your entire outlook may even be brighter with the support of quality nutrients. What to eat? Think natural and locally sourced fresh fruits, lean meats (grass-fed beef, acorn-fed pork, etc.), nuts, seeds, cold-water fish (provided that it is safe), and vegetables. Equally important is what to avoid, which could include carbohydrates, refined sugars, processed foods, alcohol, grains, legumes, tobacco, caffeine, milk, and milk products.

Doing nothing doesn't get you anywhere. What can help is taking an alternative, individualized approach to finding the underlying factors of your problems and addressing them. As a holistic practitioner, to manage chronic problems, I believe in using the support of natural remedies instead of prescribing potentially toxic drugs, and finding the root cause of your condition instead of just treating your symptoms. Now it's your turn to decide what is right for you.

A Practical Guide to Hormone Balancing

Bioidentical hormone replacement therapy (BHRT), at its core, is meant to give us the support we need to feel, look, and be younger. It is essentially meant to trick nature into believing that we're still full of life and fertile.

Once we hit the age of twenty-five, our hormones start to decline and our bodies begin preparing us for death. Although we may not think this way at that time, nature thinks we have hit our peak and is now working to clear us out to make room for the next younger and more fertile generation.

To counter that, we need to trick nature into believing that we're still vibrant and able to reproduce so that it leaves us alone to get the best out of life.

As we get closer to menopause, our hormones are all over the place. Completely unbalanced, we suffer from physical and emotional symptoms—sometimes pretty manageable, and other times so rough that they drastically affect our personal and professional lives. Hot flashes can ruin our sex lives, mood swings can destroy our jobs and families, and physical changes can leave our jobs in jeopardy. What can we do?

This is where bioidentical hormone replacement therapy comes in.

Hormone replacement might correct hormonal deficiencies and ensure optimal levels but should not go above that. It should be a balance between hormones, which means that all hormones should be checked and corrected, not just one.

Our first important question is, can hormonal replacement suppress your natural hormone production? Yes it can. If you're receiving too many hormones, your own hormonal production will be shut down. But if you are getting hormones just to correct the deficiencies, your own hormonal production will be suppressed just a little bit (no more than 30 to 40 percent) to give your own endocrine glands some rest instead of exhausting them.

The important thing is that if you take bioidentical hormones, be sure to choose the best brand and correct way to get them. And schedule regular follow-ups!

Give your hormones support by eating high-quality food. A Paleolithic diet of fruits, nuts, seeds, vegetables, meat, poultry, and fish is the best option. Avoid dairy products. They create digestive problems because of lactose; since we don't have the enzyme lactase to digest it, the lactose might remain undigested in the gut. Dairy products could cause allergies that can further damage your gut and allow contaminants to go into your bloodstream, and might also promote yeast overgrowth because of their inherent lactose. In fact, some dairy products like cheese actually contain yeast.

In addition, you might want to avoid grains because they contain carbohydrates that are not so good for the endocrine system, especially the pancreatic gland and its insulin production, and they might create weight gain. Moreover, carbohydrates might be a very good food source for yeast, so they might promote yeast overgrowth as well.

Some grains, especially wheat, also contain a protein called gluten that we might not be able to digest properly. If it goes undigested and creates inflammation of the gut, it has several possible consequences:

1. The inflammation might shut down our cognitive function—our brain—because of increased cortisol production.
2. It is linked to creating holes in the gut, allowing bad stuff like bacteria and yeast as well as toxins to go into our blood—the so-called leaky gut syndrome.
3. Inflammation requires more cortisol, which is a steroid like testosterone, estrogen, and progesterone. To make cortisol,

your body has to sacrifice the production of the above sex hormones—a phenomenon known as a cortisol steal.

Foods with a high glycemic index that raise our sugar levels too high and too fast might create a hormonal imbalance or make an existing one worse. To bring sugar levels down, our body doesn't have any choice but to suppress the production of growth hormone, testosterone,[20] progesterone,[21] and possibly estrogen. Needless to say, high-glycemic foods can undermine all your hormone replacement therapy.

Alcohol and caffeine can also pose problems. Alcohol interferes with digestion by slowing it down and also increases the activity of the enzyme aromatase that increases the conversion of testosterone into estradiol. Even if you aren't getting enough testosterone, it could be converted into estrogen.

It's very important to get enough minerals, microelements, and vitamins in your daily diet. Many enzymes have microelements in them, so if you don't have enough microelements, you don't have enough enzymes. The same applies to vitamins. Minerals are also critical because minerals like magnesium are responsible for cell electric potential. Common problems with minerals, microelements, and vitamins include not receiving enough in our food because of soil exhaustion of microelements—even though plants can still grow because of fertilizers. Even eating organic fruits and vegetables will not solve the problem.

Also, if there is a digestive problem, you may not be able to absorb vitamins, minerals, and microelements even if you consume the best-quality foods in the world. Go organic and fix your gut. If your gut isn't working properly, no matter what you eat, no matter how many supplements you take, they're going to be wasted.

Melatonin—The Hormone of Darkness

Do you suffer from menopause-related anxiety? Is it hard for you to get to sleep or stay asleep? Do you wind up fighting through every day because you're tired and can't function?

You might be melatonin deficient.

If you suffer from melatonin deficiency, you may notice that you don't sleep well and that it takes you a long time to fall asleep. You may not have a restful sleep. You may become anxious or depressed, and the change in seasons may have a more drastic effect on your emotional state.

Made in the pineal gland and about pea size, melatonin has been called the hormone of darkness—suppressed by blue light (daytime) and not suppressed by yellow light (nighttime fires).[22] First discovered in 1917, it was not named or isolated until 1958. The discovery that melatonin is an antioxidant was made in 1993.[23]

In fact, light is so important to our sleep patterns that the use of blue-blocking goggles a few hours before people go to bed has facilitated the production of melatonin to help them go to sleep.[24]

If you wear glasses that block blue light, it would be interesting to see if yellow glasses could help you go to sleep.

Melatonin is linked to helping us to go to sleep, works as an antioxidant[25] and immunomodulator,[26] increases vivid dreaming by increasing REM sleep,[27] reduces ischemic damage in experiments, improves learning and memory in experiments, possibly prevents Alzheimer's in laboratory experiments (not yet in humans), and might be linked to improved thyroid function, increased gonadotropin levels, restored fertility and menstruation, and preventing menopausal depression.[28] In cancer patients, melatonin is linked to reduced incidence of death.[29] It is even linked to weight reduction and might be linked to headache relief.[30]

Forms of treatment can include melatonin pills and sublingual drops. Warning: increasing your melatonin dose too much can actually exacerbate your problems because melatonin works optimally in very small doses.

Here might be some thoughts to boost melatonin production naturally:

- During the day, increase sunlight exposure and avoid alcohol, coffee, and smoking.

- In the evening, allow no light, noise, or electromagnetic radiation in the bedroom. Turn off computers, alarm clocks, electric devices,[31] and fuses if possible. Consider buying an electromagnetic shielded canopy.

Growth Hormone—The Body Builder

Do you have trouble losing weight? Do you feel like you have too much fat and are getting weak? Are you losing muscle mass? Do you look older than you should? Are your sex organs shrinking?

Maybe you don't have enough HGH.

HGH, or human growth hormone, is regulated by the growth hormone-releasing hormone produced in the hypothalamus. Influenced by sleep, stress, exercise, and food intake, the growth hormone-releasing hormone determines how much HGH to release into the bloodstream.[32]

While HGH does several things, it is important to know that there is a lot of controversy surrounding it. Although it is not illegal and is used for several medical conditions, the hormone is also misused in the sports world. Because it increases muscle mass, it is not allowed to be used in nearly every professional sport. And although it's not illegal, its use is very closely monitored.

HGH is linked to increasing:

- height in children
- calcium retention, thus improving bone mineralization
- muscle mass
- brain growth
- glucose production by the liver, which reduces appetite
- immune system function
- pancreatic function
- fat breakdown

HGH was most commonly used initially in children to help with height.

In adults, low HGH levels can lead to muscle mass loss, obesity, low energy, poor quality of life, hunching, thinning hair, premature aging, sex organ atrophy, poor concentration, loss of control, exhaustion, and inability to cope with stress. You eat less meat because HGH is the builder—if there is no building anymore, you do not want meat, which has muscle-building proteins.[33]

An IGF- 1 (insulin growth factor-1) test can help identify a growth hormone deficiency. While HGH levels fluctuate during daytime, the HGH level goes up mostly during sleep. Hormones that might increase HGH include thyroid hormone, DHEA, melatonin, testosterone, and estradiol.[34]

Here might be some thoughts to try to boost HGH naturally:

- Get enough sleep. Since HGH is produced mainly in the first two to three hours of sleep, go to bed when the sun goes down.
- Consume amino acids—glutamine, arginine, lysine, meats, etc.
- Eat a Paleolithic diet of organic foods.
- Maintain a low body fat while still getting enough calories.
- Avoid tobacco, street drugs, alcohol, caffeine, dairy products, and wheat, and other gluten-containing products.

In 1990, the *New England Journal of Medicine* published a study where growth hormone was used to treat a dozen men over age sixty. All of them benefited from growth hormone's antiaging wonders. A later study at the Stanford University School of Medicine showed also that it helped elderly patients. However, the article noted that they felt this was merely an increase in water since other factors like bone density and cholesterol levels were not affected.[35]

The interesting thing about this article is that it stated that the human growth hormone has multiple side effects like swelling, arthralgia, carpal tunnel syndrome, and gynecomastia, but those are symptoms of growth hormone overdose—like swelling, which is an accumulation of water. Maybe that's what they assumed happened to muscles: an increase in mass but no increase in strength? Could it be a human growth hormone overdose? So maybe just a tiny physiologic dose of growth hormone is a solution?

Thyroid Hormone—The Chief of Your Metabolism

Are you putting on too much weight or having trouble losing it? Are your thoughts not as fast as before? Is it difficult for you to get out of bed in the morning? Are you getting puffy? All of these problems indicate potentially low thyroid hormone levels.

The main thyroid hormones are T3 (the most important) and T4, which are responsible for your metabolism. Regulated by the pituitary hormone TSH, they increase energy production, blood sugar levels, fat breakdown, temperature, and heart rate. The more TSH, the more T3 and T4. T3 and T4 inhibit TSH production. A high TSH level suggests low thyroid, unless a pituitary tumor is present. To make thyroid hormones, your body needs iodine, selenium, and other microelements. If you're not eating enough iodine-rich seafood or selenium-rich foods like Brazil nuts, you might not be able to make adequate thyroid hormones.

The possible problem with conventional treatments of low thyroid, or hypothyroidism, is that monitoring usually only includes TSH instead of checking the most important acting hormone, T3. Another problem might be a medication called Synthroid, which is T4. T4 itself can inhibit TSH and make it normal. But it does not necessary mean that T4 is actually converted into T3, which is the acting thyroid hormone. The reason for this is that T4 can be converted into T3, which is an active hormone, as well as into reversed T3, which is inactive. The solution might be to take T3 and T4 in natural proportions to support your thyroid gland.

To demonstrate the bias in the official medical press, let's take a look at the article published in the most respected medical journal in the United States, the *New England Journal of Medicine*. Their study concluded that patients' satisfaction was higher when they were taking a combination of T3 and T4 than taking T4 alone. But even though it is a proven fact, almost every doctor is giving Synthroid, which is T4, and not giving T3. The funny thing is that after this article, there was an editorial[36] that concluded that both hormones (T3 and T4) aren't recommended. Doesn't making patients feel better count?

Symptoms of low thyroid include low energy, swelling, overweight, frequent ear nose and throat infections, always being cold, snoring, daytime sleepiness, no thirst, dry hair, brittle nails, bloating, joint pain, slow thoughts, and apathy.

Here might be some thoughts to boost your thyroid hormone production naturally:

- Make sure to get adequate sleep.
- Eat an organic Paleolithic diet that includes enough red meat for iron, seafood for iodine, and Brazil nuts for selenium.
- Shun processed foods, alcohol, vinegar, milk products, cereals, caffeine, and chronic stress.

Clinical Pearl: Dry palms and no hair in the outer thirds of your eyebrows are suggestive of low thyroid. Wet palms may suggest high thyroid or anxiety.

Cortisol—The Hormone of Stress

Do you have no energy at all? Are you so tired in the morning that you can't function without a cup of coffee? If the answers are yes, you may be low on the hormone cortisol.

Cortisol is made in the adrenals, the small glands just above the kidneys, and it production is stimulated by the pituitary hormone ACTH. It gives us the ability to respond to stress properly.

Excess cortisol might occur if you have too much stress or caffeine, too little sleep or estrogen, are burned out, or are using contraceptive pills. It might hurt you because too much cortisol might increase your body fat, break down your tissues (like bones), decrease your immune response (making you more susceptible to infection), and harm your memory by damaging one of the most important parts of your brain—your hippocampus. Cortisol might also decrease your sex hormone production by using cholesterol for its synthesis instead of making sex hormones (the so-called cortisol steal phenomenon). It may also decrease your serotonin production, which is responsible for your ability to adapt, by blocking conversion of tryptophan into 5 HTP and then serotonin. Too much cortisol might even cause insomnia.

On the other hand, low cortisol can make you fatigued, inflamed all over your body, and affect your sinuses, gut, throat, and so on. Low cortisol can make you very weak.

Here might be some thoughts that might give you the support you need to bring down your cortisol level if it's too high:

- magnesium (Be sure to talk to your doctor, because if you have certain medical conditions, you cannot take magnesium without a doctor's supervision.)
- laughter
- sex
- omega-3 fatty acids
- vitamin C (Consult with your physician, because if you have certain conditions, you cannot take vitamin C.)

And here might be some thoughts to increase your cortisol level:

- Get more light exposure if your doctor approves it.
- Eat frequent, small meals based on a Paleolithic diet.
- Limit or eliminate alcohol, caffeine, carbohydrates, especially simple sugars, cereals, milk, and chronic stress.

Cortisol replacement needs to be strictly monitored and should be taken exactly on time as outlined by your physician. If the time fluctuates, it can screw up your whole day/night cycle. If you're taking cortisol supplementation, you can't stop it abruptly; you have to taper cortisol down gradually. Never ever take cortisol-containing products without your physician's approval!

Clinical Pearl: Cortisol usually works very fast, and if low cortisol is a problem, you'll feel it soon after starting cortisol supplementation.

Estrogen—The Marilyn Monroe Hormone

Is your vagina so dry that sex has become a painful chore? Do you have embarrassing hot flashes all the time, or is your memory so bad now that you're afraid of making costly mistakes? Are your energy and desire going down, while your bones are getting weaker? Are you gaining weight mostly in your hip area, and you can't get rid of it no matter what you do?

Your low estrogen may be the possible reason.

Estrogen plays a critical role in the body. It's responsible for breast development, vaginal lubrication, fat burning, bone maintenance, skin and vessels, elevating good cholesterol, and bringing down bad cholesterol. Because estrogen works as an antioxidant, it protects your brain. No estrogen equals mood and memory problems.

Estrogen was also found to be responsible for women's attractiveness. That's why it is called the Marilyn Monroe hormone.[37]

There are actually three different types of estrogens: E1, E2, and E3. E2 (estradiol) is the primary and strongest estrogen produced by the ovaries and impacts more than four hundred functions in the female body. When it begins depleting naturally as women approach middle age, it can begin causing the hot flashes, mood swings, and other symptoms associated with menopause. E3 (estriol) is the weakest and might be the safest. In-vitro study suggests that estriol might be beneficial for breast cancer protection because it works as an antagonist of G protein-coupled estrogen receptor. E3 is mainly produced during pregnancy. It can provide a great support to fight vaginal dryness and as a component of bioidentical estrogen creams. E1 (estrone) might be linked to carcinogenesis and is therefore rarely used.

Here are some thoughts that might give you the support you need to increase your estrogen naturally:

- Lose weight.
- Avoid chronic stress.
- Be sure to get enough calories from an organic food-based Paleolithic diet.
- Steer clear of carbohydrates, cereals, caffeine, and milk. Limit other dairy products as well, as the estrogen and progesterone levels in cows when they're milked are extremely high.
- Curtail smoking, marijuana, and other street drugs.

To see if you have an increased risk of cancer because of estrogen, have some lab work done. You need to figure out how your body is disposing of estrogen. It's fine if your body is doing it right, but it can harm you if your body cannot dispose of estrogen properly.

Clinical Pearl: Decreased vaginal moisture is suggestive of low estrogen level. Usually the vagina is wet if you have enough estrogen. Having enough estrogen is indicated by full breasts, a low waist-to-hip ratio, and a strong desire for sex. It was often called the Marilyn Monroe hormone.

Progesterone—The Hormone of Calmness

Are you anxious all the time or finding you can't control yourself? Are you yelling more at your children and spouse? Is it tough to get a good night's sleep? Your low progesterone level might the problem.

Progesterone can help balance confidence and strong sexual desire and can also calm you down. Most pregnant women are calm because they have plenty of progesterone.

Progesterone naturally produced in your body also normalizes blood pressure and works as a natural diuretic and antidepressant. Its main job is to balance estrogen.

Here might be some thoughts to give you the support you need to increase progesterone:

- Stay away from nonorganic meat, adhesives, car exhaust, and almost all plastics.
- Ensure your body is getting adequate calories from a natural Paleolithic diet.
- Lose weight.
- Diminish stress.
- Eschew sugar, cereals, caffeine, and milk.
- Reduce or end consumption of smoking, marijuana, and other street drugs.

Low progesterone is usually indicated by poor sleep, bloating, and swelling. Progesterone supplement might be a natural sleeping support.

When your progesterone level is normalized, you'll get the support you need to feel calmer, lose weight, and improve your sleep. And you and your spouse will be happier! Don't use any over-the-counter progesterone-containing products without consulting your doctor.

Testosterone—The Rejuvenating Elixir

Do you have no sex drive? Too many wrinkles or "chicken hands"? No more energy? Then maybe your low testosterone level is a problem.

There should be something that gives us energy and a sense of well-being, as well as ability to maintain our muscles, mental and muscle energy, and libido. It is the hormone testosterone that does the job.

Testosterone is not only tasked with your sex drive, erections, and muscles. It also is linked to maintaining your bones and protecting you from diabetes, Alzheimer's, heart disease, and other ailments.

Low testosterone can cause a low sex drive, mood problems, fatigue, and sleep issues.

Here might be some thoughts to give you the support you need to raise your testosterone levels:

- Attain and maintain a healthy weight.
- Eat foods high in protein and relatively low in carbs.

- Be more active.
- Pick your produce by consuming plenty of fruits and vegetables.
- Avoid chronic stress.
- Strive for quality, uninterrupted sleep.
- Optimize your calories by eating a Paleolithic diet rich in organic foods.
- Steer clear of sugar, cereals, caffeine, and milk.
- Keep away from alcohol, smoking, marijuana, and other street drugs.
- Men could benefit from avoiding tight underwear and hot baths to reduce testicles temperature.

Low testosterone is usually suggested by a low libido, wrinkles, and a jawline drop. A classic sign might be "chicken hands."

Clinical Pearl: If you're using testosterone cream, rotate the sites to avoid excessive hair growth.

FSH and LH—The Hormones of Reproduction

Have you been trying to get pregnant for a while, with no success? If all other factors have been ruled out, it might be time to take a look at your follicle-stimulating hormone (FSH) and luteinizing hormone (LH) levels.

Working in tandem, FSH and LH play vital roles in the reproductive process.[38] In women, they help regulate the menstrual cycle and egg production by the ovaries—fluctuating throughout the monthly cycle, and at their zenith right before ovulation. For LH, this is known as an "LH surge."

In men, FSH and LH have equally important parts to play as they're charged with testosterone and sperm production.

Prolactin—The "Got Milk?" Hormone

Have you noticed how much your breasts swell when you're pregnant? Do they feel tender to the touch? Chances are, it's because your milk is coming in—thanks to the hormone prolactin.

Used to make breast milk, prolactin levels surge by ten to twenty times during pregnancy and remain elevated if you breastfeed your baby.[39] They tend to be highest during sleep or upon awakening and can also increase when you're emotionally or physically stressed.

DHEA—The Sex Hormone Producer

As you've gotten older, have you found yourself gaining weight and losing enthusiasm for life?

Some experts suggest that DHEA might be the answer.

Dehydroepiandrosterone (DHEA) is a mouthful but has a pivotal impact on the male and female reproductive system. Produced in the adrenal glands, intestine, and liver, DHEA is charged with the production of sex hormones—estrogens in women and androgens in men.[40] While DHEA levels begin decreasing after age thirty for both genders, the rate is more rapid for women.

Some experts suggest that DHEA could be used to treat depression, obesity, and osteoporosis, with the verdict still out on its effects on sexual function, lupus, and hormonal disorders. However, there are no controlled studies yet. [43]

Oxytocin—The Hormone of Love

Wonder what the hormone is that puts you in the mood for love? Affectionately referred to by such varying monikers as the "hug hormone," "cuddle chemical," "moral molecule," and "bliss hormone," oxytocin gets its romantic reputation due to its effect on love and the female reproductive process.[41]

Made in the hypothalamus of the brain, oxytocin not only induces feelings of love but also regulates two critical aspects of the continued propagation of our species. During labor, as the cervix and uterus widen, oxytocin is released to help the uterus muscles contract. After the baby is born, stimulation of the nipples causes further oxytocin to be produced, which helps milk production for breastfeeding.

Adrenaline and Noradrenaline—The Fight-or-Flight Hormones

Have you read stories about mothers who lifted entire cars to free their children trapped underneath? Those types of seemingly herculean feats can be credited to the presence of two hormones: adrenaline (also known as epinephrine) and noradrenaline (norephinephrine).[42]

Both hormones are triggered during stressful situations, galvanizing the body for immediate, decisive action. By increasing alertness and blood pressure, and heightening focus and memory retrieval, adrenaline and noradrenaline enable the body to perform at optimal levels during times of heightened fear, anger, or anxiety.

PMS—Premenstrual Syndrome

Are you moody and irritable during your cycle? Bloated and fatigued? Do you get overemotional and depressed?

Premenstrual syndrome, or PMS, might be the result of either low progesterone or a relatively high level of estrogen in the second part of your cycle. The latter may be due to your gut's inability to dispose of estrogen properly, or an influx of estrogen-like toxins from outside that are endocrine disruptors. Or you just might not have enough progesterone. To help rectify this imbalance, first fix your gut and then eat organic, avoid contact with plastic (including food and water containers), and decrease your weight, because some estrogen is made in fat tissue. If it doesn't work, you might consider a progesterone supplementation under your doctor's supervision.

Endometriosis

Do you suffer from painful periods or cramping? Is sex painful? Are you irritable? Like PMS, endometriosis might be linked to low progesterone or high estrogen or both. Either way, it needs to be balanced.

After first fixing your gut, some natural ways to balance your hormones might include eating organic, avoiding contact with plastic (including through your food and water), and decreasing your weight because some estrogen is made in fat tissue. If it doesn't work, then you may need a progesterone supplementation. Never ever take any progesterone-containing products without consulting your doctor, and never try to manage endometriosis on your own.

Uterine Fibroids

Uterine fibroids are benign muscle tumors that originate from the uterus. Their growth is dependent on the estrogen-progesterone balance. Fibroid management is based on restoration of the proper estrogen-progesterone ratio and is practically the same as PMS management.

Uterine fibroids may require surgery if not controlled by conservative measures.

Ovarian Cysts

Do you have uncomfortable ovarian cysts? Do you experience pain during periods? Spotting? Are you nauseous or vomiting?

Ovarian cysts can be due to several reasons that include enlarged follicles, leftover tissue, cancer, and benign tumors. There are several types of cysts as well. Never try to manage ovarian cysts on your own because they might be malignant.

You might try to naturally prevent and treat ovarian cysts by eating organic, avoiding contact with plastic (including through your food and water), and decreasing your weight because some estrogen is made in fat tissue. If it doesn't work, then you may need progesterone supplementation. Needless to say, all of the above should be done only under your doctor's supervision.

Benign Prostatic Hypertrophy—BPH

Are you getting up to go to the bathroom often? Is your stream weak? When you have to urinate, are you unable to hold it in?

Benign prostatic hypertrophy is an increase in the size of the prostate. The symptoms are uncomfortable pain and an increase in the urge and frequency of urination. It is important to get your prostate checked regularly. Never try to manage prostate problems on your own.

Here might be some thoughts to get prostate support naturally:

- Decrease your body weight, because your fat and muscles are where testosterone is converted into estrogen, which stimulates prostate growth.
- Drink pomegranate juice.
- Avoid caffeine and alcohol.
- Saw Palmetto might also beneficial, as well as fish oil.

Toxins—The Hormone Disruptors

In 1970, biologist Mike Gilbertson observed an unusually high death rate among gull chicks in Lake Ontario. Not only did many of them die before hatching, but they also had a huge amount of unusual body and body-part shapes. It finally occurred to him that he had seen similar abnormalities in dioxine-poisoned chicks. His colleagues practically laughed at him; after all, there was no dioxide in Lake Ontario.

Ten years later, fishermen in the United States and Canada noticed a declining salmon population due to too many females and too few males. Scientists found no problems with the male-to-female ratio after hatching, but when they checked the ratio down the river, females vastly outnumbered males. What happened to the males? It remained a mystery until they decided to check the salmons' genes.

Astonishingly enough, gene analysis suggested that there were no problems with genes: the male-to-female ratio was about 1:1. But while going down the river, the males had become females. After ruling out other factors, the scientists attributed this sex reversal to exposure to man-made compounds like pesticides and detergents that worked like environmental estrogens.

Fast forward ten more years to the Great Lakes. Theo Colborn, a professor of zoology at the University of Florida, Gainesville, noticed something unusual—nest building by two females. It was highly unusual. Suspecting a hormonal influence, she started studying endocrinology herself after her endocrinology colleagues expressed no interest. Colborn discovered that the Swedish toxicologist Bengtsson was concerned with the shrinkage of fish reproductive organs due to organochlorine compound-tainted Baltic water. Could it be a hormone disruption?

In 1991, Colburn gathered scientists to discuss the findings about gender alterations secondary to environmental toxins that behave like hormones. They issued a document called the "Wingspread Consensus Statement," coining the terms "endocrine disruption" and "endocrine disruptors."

Toxins have a deleterious effect on our hormones. Mercury, for example, inhibits adrenaline breakdown by blocking the enzyme catecholamine O methyl transferase, which results in anxiety, palpitations. and high blood pressure. Lead toxicity is known to cause decreased libido. Endocrine disruptors, especially environmental estrogens, were linked to multiple problems, including cancer.[44] If you suspect that you might have increased toxins levels, don't try to do detoxification on your own. Find a doctor who specializes in this area.

In Conclusion

Now that we know more about hormones, let's ask some of the same questions we posed before:

- Is it hard for you to get to sleep or stay asleep?
- Do you have no more energy at all?
- Are you putting on too much weight or having trouble losing it?
- Do you find yourself yelling more at your children and spouse?
- Are you having embarrassing hot flashes?
- Is your sex drive lacking?

If you answered yes to any of the above questions—especially if you're middle-aged or older—it's time to have a frank conversation with your physician about your hormones.

Hormones play pivotal roles in our bodies. They regulate our sleep, growth, metabolism, energy levels, and reproductive systems. They help us feel calm and position us for quick response during stressful times. And that's not even taking into account what they do for our sex lives—lubricating the vagina, causing erections, and putting both men and women in the proper mood for love.

Sometimes people wonder whether they should take synthetic hormones.

What I tell them is that it is their responsibility to decide and that they should not make any health decision without consulting their doctor.

What I usually tell myself, and only myself, is this: if in doubt, think natural.

As an illustration, there's probably nothing more natural than going to the bathroom. It's not something we talk about a lot, but most of us think that the proper technique is sitting on a toilet and letting gravity take its course. What most of us don't realize is that that's not the way nature intended us to defecate—and that we really should be squatting to avoid undue strain to the body. When we squat, our knees are closer to our torso, which might help maximize elimination efficiencies while minimizing the risks of constipation, hemorrhoids, and other bowel or pelvic complications. Squatting may not be for everyone, but it's natural and something that I do to help keep my body in proper balance.

Which brings us back to the synthetic versus bioidentical hormones discussion. It is my understanding that even a small tweak in one area may unintentionally cause a much larger, potentially disastrous ramification in another area. Altering hormones might be like tossing a pebble into a pond, with the ensuing ripples being more far-reaching than we ever imagined. If that's the case, it may seem to make sense to start from something that is closer to a natural substance rather than a man-made one. This is just a thought, not an endorsement. As with anything health related, it's really up to the individual and his or her doctor to determine the best course of action.

Keep in mind that bioidentical hormones are still hormones with their inherent risks and benefits. And so far, there is no proof that bioidentical hormones are safer than their synthetic counterparts. Long-term, controlled, randomized studies would be needed to prove or disprove that bioidentical hormones are safer, but no such studies have been done so far or are planned for the future. And we may never have them because of lack of funding.

If any of your hormones are out of balance, it can cause your entire life to be out of balance as well. Don't you deserve to live a happy, healthy, and productive life, feeling—and looking—as young as possible?

Bioidentical hormone replacement might give you the support you need to get your life back.

Dr. Kalitenko Bio

Doctor Kalitenko is board-certified in internal medicine, with offices in Brooklyn (718-382-9200) and Great Neck (516-467-0253), New York. Throughout his career as a medical doctor, he has supported many patients by providing personalized care and leveraging the most current traditional and holistic medicine therapies.

After graduating from Donetsk Medical Institute in the Ukraine at age twenty-one, Dr. Kalitenko served as an emergency care physician and later became head of the Hyperbaric Oxygenation Department of the Donetsk Clinical Hospital in Donetsk, Ukraine.

Upon moving to the United States, Dr. Kalitenko finished his medical residency in Brooklyn, New York, was board-certified in internal medicine, and became a staff physician at a teaching hospital to support both inpatient and outpatient care. In 2001, he decided he could better serve patients through his own practice, utilizing a functional and holistic approach to traditional medicine. His philosophy is simple: identify the root causes of patients' unique concerns and address them as naturally as possible, promoting a healthy lifestyle and overall wellness.

For more information about Dr. Kalitenko's services, visit www. kalitenko.com. For medical news, read his blog at http://www.kalitenko. com/blog or sign up for valuable e-seminars that can help you achieve your health goals in a natural way.

Disclaimer

The content in this book reflects Dr. Sergey Kalitenko's personal philosophy and approach to practicing safe, responsible medicine and has been provided for informational purposes only. Any patients referenced have had their stories modified to protect their privacy.

Please note that Dr. Kalitenko's suggestions should not be misconstrued as health statements, nor are they intended to substitute for medical advice. His thoughts are for information purposes only and should not be interpreted as an advice to help, treat, alleviate or cure any disease or symptoms. As with anything regarding your health, it's necessary to talk with your doctor before making any health decisions that might impact your overall well-being.

In addition, the above opinions do not reflect those of the American Boards of Medical Professions, Food and Drug Administration, or other government agencies. It is also critical to note that not all bioidentical hormones are FDA approved, and their use is not routinely recommended by organizations like the International Menopause Society, American Medical Association, American College of Obstetricians and Gynecologists, Mayo Clinic, Endocrine Society, and so on.

References

1   N. Singer, "Menopause, as Brought to You by Big Pharma," *New York Times* (12 December, 2009).

2   (25 February, 2016), Troglitazone, *Wikipedia.*

3   (29 February, 2016), Trovafloxacin, *Wikipedia.*

4   N. Singer, "Medical Papers by Ghostwriters Pushed Therapy," *New York Times* (4 August, 2009).

5   (2010), WHI Postmenopausal Hormone Therapy Trials, NHBLI Women's Health Initiative.

6   (2010), WHI Postmenopausal Hormone Therapy Trials, NHBLI Women's Health Initiative.

7   P. Smith, "A comprehensive look at hormones and the effects of hormone replacement." 14th Annual International Congress on Anti-Aging Medicine, Orlando, FL., Vol. 5., retrieved June (2005).

8   "Plasma Lipid and Lipoprotein Pattern in Greenlandic West-Coast Eskimos," *Lancet* 297, no. 7710: 1143–1146.

9   "Kavita Study," http://www.staffanlindeberg.com.

10 (19 December, 2015), "Grandmother Hypothesis," *Wikipedia.*

11 (19 December, 2015), "Patriarch Hypothesis," *Wikipedia.*

12 (19 December, 2015), "Estradiol," *Wikipedia.*

13 (23 March, 2015), "Estrogen," *Wikipedia.*

14 (1 March, 2015), "Milk." *Wikipedia.*

15 (17 March, 2016), "Testosterone," *Wikipedia.*

16 (17 March, 2016), "Testosterone," *Wikipedia.*

17 AD Marcus, "Chronic-Fatigue Link to Virus Disputed," *Wall Street Journal* (30 June, 2010).

18 K Holtorf, "The bioidentical hormone debate: are bioidentical hormones (estradiol, estriol, and progesterone) safer or more efficacious than commonly used synthetic versions in hormone replacement therapy?" *Postgraduate Medicine* 121.1 (2009): 73–85.

19   C. Derzko, "Bioidentical Hormone Therapy at Menopause" (pdf), *Endocrinology Rounds* 9, no. 6 (2009): 1–6.

20   (14 June, 2009), "Testosterone Decreases after Ingestion of Sugar," The Endocrine Society.

21   MY Mei-Po and MMP Yang, "Effect of a Single Dose of Progesterone on Blood Glucose in Rats," *Endocrine Society* (1 July, 2013).

22   GC Brainard, JP Hanifin, JM Greeson, B Byrne, G Glickman, E Gerner, Rollag, "Action spectrum for melatonin regulation in humans: evidence for a novel circadian photoreceptor," *J Neurosci.* 15;21, no. 16 (August 15, 2001): 6405–12, PMID 11487664.

L Kayumov, RF Casper, RJ Hawa, B Perelman, SA Chung, S Sokalsky, Shipiro, "Blocking low-wavelength light prevents nocturnal melatonin suppression with no adverse effect on performance during simulated shift work," *J Clin Endocrinol Metab.* 90, no. 5 (May 2005): 2755–61, doi:10.1210/jc.2004-2062, PMID 15713707.

23   Paul M. Coates, *Encyclopedia of Dietary Supplements*, Marc R. Blackman, Gordon M. Cragg, Mark Levine, Joel Moss, Jeffrey D. White (CRC Press, 2005), 457–466, ISBN 0824755049, retrieved 2009-03-31.

AM Filadelfi, AM Castrucci, "Comparative aspects of the pineal/melatonin system of poikilothermic vertebrates," *Journal of Pineal Research* 20, no. 4 (May 1996): 175–86, doi:10.1111/j.1600-079X.1996.tb00256.x. PMID 8836950.

AM Filadelfi, AM Castrucci, "Comparative aspects of the pineal/melatonin system of poikilothermic vertebrates," *Journal of Pineal Research* 20, no. 4 (May 1996): 175–86, doi:10.1111/j.1600-079X.1996.tb00256.x. PMID 8836950.

AB Lerner, JD Case, Y Takahashi, "Isolation of melatonin and 5-methoxyindole-3-acetic acid from bovine pineal glands," *J Biol Chem* 235 (1960): 1992–7, PMID 14415935.

HJ Lynch, RJ Wurtman, MA Moskowitz, MC Archer, MH Ho, "Daily rhythm in human urinary melatonin," *Science* 187, no. 4172 (January 1975): 169–71, doi:10.1126/science.1167425. PMID 1167425.

D.X. Tan, "Melatonin: a potent, endogenous hydroxyl radical scavenger," *Endocr J* 1 (1993): 57–60.

24   GC Brainard, JP Hanifin, JM Greeson, B Byrne, G Glickman, E Gerner, Rollag, "Action spectrum for melatonin regulation in humans: evidence for a novel circadian photoreceptor," *J Neurosci.* 15;21, no. 16 (August 15, 2001): 6405–12, PMID 11487664.

L Kayumov, RF Casper, RJ Hawa, B Perelman, SA Chung, S Sokalsky, Shipiro, "Blocking low-wavelength light prevents nocturnal melatonin suppression with no adverse effect on performance during simulated shift work," *J Clin Endocrinol Metab.* 90, no. 5 (May 2005): 2755–61, doi:10.1210/jc.2004-2062, PMID 15713707.

25 D.X. Tan, "Melatonin: a potent, endogenous hydroxyl radical scavenger," *Endocr J* 1 (1993): 57–60.

26 A Carrillo-Vico, J Guerrero, P Lardone, R Reiter, "A review of the multiple actions of melatonin on the immune system," *Endocrine* 27 no. 2 (2005): 189–200, doi:10.1385/ENDO:27:2:189. PMID 16217132.
    E Arushanian, E Beier, "Immunotropic properties of pineal melatonin," *Eksp Klin Farmakol* 65, no. 5 (2002): 73–80. PMID 12596522.

27 Alan Lewis, *Melatonin and the Biological Clock* (McGraw-Hill, 1999), 23, ISBN 0879837349.

28 G Bellipanni, F Di Marzo, F Blasi, A Di Marzo, "Effects of melatonin in perimenopausal and menopausal women: our personal experience," *Ann N Y Acad Sci* 1057 (Dec. 2005): 393–402, doi:10.1196/annals.1356.030. PMID 16399909.

29 E Mills, P Wu, D Seely, G. E. Guyatt, P Wu, D Seely, G Guyatt, "Melatonin in the treatment of cancer: a systematic review of randomized controlled trials and meta-analysis," *Journal of pineal research* 39, no. 4 (2005): 360, doi:10.1111/j.1600-079X.2005.00258.x. PMID 16207291.

30 J Barrenetxe, P Delagrange, J Martínez, "Physiological and metabolic functions of melatonin," *J Physiol Biochem* 60, no. 1 (2004): 61–72, doi:10.1007/BF03168221, PMID 15352385.

31 D Dodick, D Capobianco, "Treatment and management of cluster headache," *Curr Pain Headache Rep* 5, no. 1 (2001): 83–91, doi:10.1007/s11916-001-0015-0, PMID 11252143.
    J Gagnier, "The therapeutic potential of melatonin in migraines and other headache types," *Altern Med Rev* 6, no. 4 (2001): 383–9, PMID 11578254.

32 (12 December, 2014), "Growth hormone-releasing hormone." http://www.yourhormones.info.

33 Thierry Hertoghe, MD, *The Hormone Handbook* (International medical Books).

34 D Rudman, AG Feller, HS Nagraj, GA Gergans, PY Lalitha, AF Goldberg, RA Schlenker, L Cohn, IW Rudman, DE Mattson, "Effects of human growth hormone in men over 60 years old," *N. Engl. J. Med.* 323, no. 1 (July 1990): 1–6, PMID 2355952.
    H Liu, DM Bravata, Olkin I, S Nayak, B Roberts, AM Garber, AR Hoffman, "Systematic review: the safety and efficacy of growth hormone in the healthy elderly," *Ann. Intern. Med.* 146, no. 2 (January 2007): 104–15, PMID 17227934.
    "No proof that growth hormone therapy makes you live longer, study finds," PhysOrg.com, 2007-01-16, retrieved 2009-03-16.
    Mark L Gordon, MD, Human Growth Hormone (HGH) as an Anti-Aging Agent.
    Alex Kuczynski, "Anti-Aging Potion or Poison?" *New York Times* (12 April, 1998).

35 Daniel Rudman, MD, Axel G. Feller, MD, Hoskote S. Nagraj, MD, Gregory A. Gergans, MD, Pardee Y. Lalitha, MD, Allen F. Goldberg, DDS, Robert A. Schlenker, PhD, Lester Cohn, MD, Inge W. Rudman, BS, and Dale E. Mattson, PhD, "Effects of Human Growth Hormone in Men over 60 Years Old," *N Engl J Med* 323 (5 July, 1990): 1-6.

36 Robertas Bunevičius, MD, PhD, Gintautas Kažanavičius, MD, PhD, Rimas Žalinkevičius, MD, and Arthur J. Prange Jr., MD, "Effects of Thyroxine as Compared with Thyroxine plus Triiodothyronine in Patients with Hypothyroidism," *N Engl J Med* 340 (11 February, 1999):424–429.

37 E Callaway, "High hormone levels in women linked to unfaithfulness," https://www.newscientist.com (14 January, 2009).

38 (2014), "Follicle-Stimulating Hormone," *WebMD.com*.

39 (2014), "Prolactin," *WebMD.com*.

40 (2014), "Drugs and Supplements DHEA," Natural Standard Research Collaboration.

41 M MacGill, "Oxytocin: What is it and what does it do?" *Medical News Today* (21 September, 2015).

42 Adrenaline, http://medical-dictionary.thefreedictionary.com/ (24 March, 2016), Norepinephrine, *Wikipedia*.

43 (16 June, 2015), "DHEA," National Institutes of Health.

44 Harrison, P. T. C., Humfrey, C. D. N., Litchfield, M., Peakall, D., & Shuker, L. K., IEH assessment on environmental oestrogens: Consequences to human health and wildlife, (Leicester, UK: MRC Institute for Environment and Health, 1995).

Printed in Great Britain
by Amazon

41613078R00037